Title: The Amazing World of Protein

Subtitle: A Comprehensive Guide

Author: Marcel Soppart

Book Description:

Discover the importance of protein in this comprehensive guide tailored for all readers. "The Amazing World of Protein" provides detailed explanations, practical insights, and essential knowledge about protein. Learn how this crucial nutrient supports growth, health, and daily activities through in-depth chapters and clear, factual content.

Table of Contents:

Chapter 1: Introduction to Protein

What is Protein?

Protein is a vital nutrient made up of long chains of amino acids. These amino acids are the building blocks of all cells in the human body. Protein plays a crucial role in the growth, repair, and maintenance of tissues. Unlike carbohydrates and fats, the body does not store protein, so it needs to be consumed regularly through diet.

The Structure of Protein

Proteins are complex molecules composed of carbon, hydrogen, oxygen, nitrogen, and sometimes sulfur. They are made up of smaller units called amino acids, which are linked together in long chains. The sequence of these amino acids determines the specific function and structure of each protein.

Protein Functions

Proteins serve a wide range of functions in the body, including:

- Structural: Providing support in tissues such as skin, hair, and muscles.

- Enzymatic: Acting as enzymes to catalyze biochemical reactions.

- Regulatory: Regulating physiological processes as hormones.

- Transport: Transporting molecules across cell membranes and through the bloodstream.

- Protective: Defending the body against pathogens as antibodies.

- Storage: Storing nutrients and ions for future use.

Protein Turnover

The body constantly breaks down and synthesizes proteins in a process known as protein turnover. This process allows the body to adapt to changing physiological conditions, repair damaged tissues, and replace old proteins.

Chapter 2: The Importance of Protein

Growth and Development

Protein is essential for growth and development, particularly during childhood, adolescence, and pregnancy. It provides the building blocks for new tissues and is crucial for the development of muscles, organs, and the immune system.

Muscle Maintenance and Repair

Protein supports muscle maintenance and repair. During physical activity, muscle fibers experience microscopic damage. Protein helps repair these fibers, leading to muscle growth and increased strength. Adequate protein intake is vital for athletes and individuals engaging in regular exercise.

Immune Function

Proteins play a key role in the immune system. Antibodies, which are proteins, identify and neutralize pathogens such as bacteria and viruses. Additionally, proteins are involved in the production of immune cells that protect the body from infections.

Hormone Production

Proteins are involved in the production of hormones that regulate various physiological processes. For example, insulin, a protein hormone, regulates blood sugar levels, while thyroid hormones control metabolism.

Enzyme Activity

Enzymes, which are proteins, catalyze biochemical reactions in the body. These reactions are essential for digestion, metabolism, and cellular functions. Without enzymes, these processes would occur too slowly to sustain life.

Energy Source

While carbohydrates and fats are the primary energy sources, protein can also be used for energy, especially during prolonged physical activity or when carbohydrate intake is insufficient. However, using protein for energy can compromise its other vital functions.

Chapter 3: Understanding Amino Acids

What are Amino Acids?

Amino acids are organic compounds that combine to form proteins. There are 20 different amino acids that the body needs to function properly. These amino acids can be classified into three categories:

- Essential amino acids: Must be obtained through diet as the body cannot synthesize them.

- Non-essential amino acids: Can be synthesized by the body.

- Conditional amino acids: Usually not essential except in times of illness and stress.

Essential Amino Acids

The nine essential amino acids are:

1. Histidine: Important for growth and repair of tissues.

2. Isoleucine: Aids in muscle metabolism and immune function.

3. Leucine: Stimulates muscle protein synthesis.

4. Lysine: Crucial for protein synthesis, hormone production, and enzyme function.

5. Methionine: Necessary for tissue growth and repair.

6. Phenylalanine: Precursor for neurotransmitters.

7. Threonine: Supports immune function and fat metabolism.

8. Tryptophan: Precursor for serotonin, which regulates mood and sleep.

9. Valine: Promotes muscle growth and tissue repair.

Non-Essential Amino Acids

The non-essential amino acids are:

1. Alanine: Plays a role in glucose metabolism.

2. Arginine: Supports immune function and wound healing.

3. Asparagine: Involved in nitrogen metabolism.

4. Aspartic acid: Participates in the citric acid cycle.

5. Cysteine: Important for protein structure and function.

6. Glutamic acid: Acts as a neurotransmitter.

7. Glutamine: Supports gut health and immune function.

8. Glycine: Involved in the synthesis of collagen and other proteins.

9. Proline: Essential for collagen production.

10. Serine: Participates in metabolic processes.

11. Tyrosine: Precursor for neurotransmitters and hormones.

Conditional Amino Acids

Conditional amino acids are usually not essential except in times of illness and stress. These include:

1. Arginine: Important for immune function during illness.

2. Cysteine: Necessary for protein synthesis during stress.

3. Glutamine: Supports immune function and gut health during

illness.

4. Tyrosine: Required for neurotransmitter production during stress.

Functions of Amino Acids

Amino acids play a critical role in various bodily functions, such as:

- Histidine: Vital for hemoglobin production.

- Isoleucine: Supports energy production and muscle recovery.

- Leucine: Regulates blood sugar levels and aids in wound healing.

- Lysine: Promotes calcium absorption and collagen formation.

- Methionine: Acts as an antioxidant and supports liver function.

- Phenylalanine: Converts to tyrosine, which is necessary for brain function.

- Threonine: Maintains protein balance and supports central nervous system function.

- Tryptophan: Converts to niacin, which is essential for metabolism.

- Valine: Supports cognitive function and emotional calmness.

Chapter 4: The History of Protein Research

Early Discoveries

The study of protein dates back to the early 19th century. In 1838, the Dutch chemist Gerardus Johannes Mulder first described proteins, naming them from the Greek word "proteios," meaning "primary" or "first place." This emphasized their importance in living organisms.

Development of Protein Chemistry

In the late 19th and early 20th centuries, scientists began to understand the chemical structure of proteins. Emil Fischer, a German chemist, made significant contributions by elucidating the peptide bond and demonstrating that proteins are composed of amino acids linked together.

Advances in Protein Structure

The mid-20th century saw major breakthroughs in understanding protein structure. Linus Pauling and Robert Corey discovered the alpha-helix and beta-sheet structures, fundamental elements of protein secondary structure. In 1958, John Kendrew and Max Perutz determined the three-dimensional structure of myoglobin and hemoglobin, respectively, using X-ray crystallography.

The Central Dogma of Molecular Biology

In the 1950s, Francis Crick and James Watson proposed the central dogma of molecular biology, which describes the flow of genetic information from DNA to RNA to protein. This discovery was pivotal in understanding how proteins are synthesized in cells.

Protein Folding and Misfolding

In the late 20th and early 21st centuries, research focused on protein folding and misfolding. Understanding how proteins fold into their functional three-dimensional shapes and how misfolding can lead to diseases such as Alzheimer's and Parkinson's has been a significant area of study.

Proteomics and Modern Protein Research

Today, proteomics—the large-scale study of proteins—plays a

crucial role in biomedical research. Advanced techniques such as mass spectrometry and bioinformatics allow scientists to analyze the proteome, the complete set of proteins expressed in a cell or organism, leading to new insights into health and disease.

Chapter 5: Complete vs. Incomplete Proteins

Complete Proteins

Complete proteins contain all nine essential amino acids in sufficient quantities. These are primarily found in animal-based foods such as meat, fish, poultry, eggs, and dairy products. Some plant-based foods like quinoa and soy are also complete proteins.

Incomplete Proteins

Incomplete proteins lack one or more

of the essential amino acids. Most plant-based proteins fall into this category. However, by combining different plant foods, you can create a complete protein. For example, eating rice and beans together provides all the essential amino acids.

Complementary Proteins

Combining two or more incomplete protein sources to provide all essential amino acids is known as complementary protein pairing. This strategy is important for vegetarians and vegans to ensure they receive adequate nutrition.

Examples of Complementary Protein Pairing

- Grains and Legumes: Rice and beans, wheat bread and peanut butter.

- Legumes and Seeds: Lentils and sunflower seeds, chickpeas and sesame seeds.

- Grains and Dairy: Oatmeal and milk, pasta with cheese.

Protein Quality

Protein quality refers to the ability of a protein source to provide all essential amino acids and support growth and maintenance. High-quality proteins are easily digestible and contain all essential amino acids in the right proportions.

Protein Digestibility-Corrected Amino Acid Score (PDCAAS)

PDCAAS is a method used to evaluate the protein quality of food based on its amino acid composition and digestibility. It ranges from 0 to 1, with 1 indicating the highest protein quality. Animal proteins typically have higher PDCAAS scores compared to plant proteins.

Biological Value (BV)

Biological Value (BV) measures the proportion of absorbed protein that becomes incorporated into the proteins of the organism's body. BV is a useful measure of protein quality, with higher values indicating better utilization by the body.

Net Protein Utilization (NPU)

Net Protein Utilization (NPU) measures the percentage of dietary protein that is retained in the body for growth and maintenance. It is calculated by comparing the nitrogen content of the protein consumed to the nitrogen content retained by the body.

Chapter 6: Sources of Protein

Animal-Based Protein Sources

1. Meat: Beef, pork, lamb
2. Poultry: Chicken, turkey, duck
3. Fish and Seafood: Salmon, tuna, shrimp, scallops
4. Eggs: Whole eggs, egg whites
5. Dairy Products: Milk, cheese, yogurt

Plant-Based Protein Sources

1. Legumes: Beans, lentils, chickpeas
2. Nuts and Seeds: Almonds, peanuts, chia seeds, sunflower seeds
3. Grains: Quinoa, brown rice, oats
4. Soy Products: Tofu, tempeh, edamame
5. Vegetables: Broccoli, spinach, Brussels sprouts

Protein Content in Common Foods

- Chicken breast (100g): 31g protein
- Salmon (100g): 25g protein
- Eggs (one large): 6g protein
- Lentils (1 cup cooked): 18g protein
- Quinoa (1 cup cooked): 8g protein

Bioavailability of Protein Sources

Bioavailability refers to how well the body can absorb and use a nutrient. Animal proteins generally have higher bioavailability compared to plant proteins due to their complete amino acid profile and ease of digestion.

High-Protein Foods and Their Benefits

1. Chicken Breast: Lean source of high-quality protein, low in fat.

2. Salmon: Rich in omega-3 fatty acids and high-quality protein.

3. Eggs: Versatile, nutrient-dense, and an excellent source of protein.

4. Lentils: High in protein and fiber, supports digestive health.

5. Quinoa: Complete protein source, gluten-free, and rich in minerals.

Factors Affecting Protein Quality

1. Amino Acid Composition: Presence of all essential amino acids in the right proportions.

2. Digestibility: The extent to which the protein is broken down and absorbed by the body.

3. Anti-Nutritional Factors: Compounds such as phytates and tannins in plant foods that can reduce protein digestibility.

Enhancing Protein Absorption

1. Cooking: Cooking methods like boiling and steaming can improve protein digestibility.

2. Fermentation: Fermenting foods like soybeans (e.g., tempeh) can enhance protein availability.

3. Soaking and Sprouting: Soaking and sprouting legumes and

grains can reduce anti-nutritional factors and improve protein absorption.

Chapter 7: Animal Proteins

Nutritional Benefits

Animal proteins are considered high-quality proteins because they contain all essential amino acids. They are also rich in other nutrients such as vitamin B12, iron, zinc, and omega-3 fatty acids.

Common Animal Protein Sources

- Meat: Red meat is a rich source of protein and iron but should be consumed in moderation due to its saturated fat content.

- Poultry: Lean poultry like chicken and turkey is a lower-fat option for protein.

- Fish and Seafood: Fish is an excellent source of protein and omega-3 fatty acids, which are beneficial for heart health.

- Dairy: Dairy products provide protein along with calcium and vitamin D, which are important for bone health.

Health Considerations

While animal proteins offer many benefits, it's important to choose lean cuts and avoid processed meats to reduce the intake of unhealthy fats and preservatives.

Environmental Impact

The production of animal proteins has a significant environmental impact, including greenhouse gas emissions, land use, and water consumption. Choosing sustainably sourced animal proteins can help mitigate these effects.

Ethical Considerations

Ethical considerations related to animal welfare and sustainable farming practices are important factors to consider when choosing animal protein sources.

Red Meat and Health

Red meat is a rich source of protein, iron, and vitamin B12. However, high consumption of red meat, especially processed red meat, has been associated with an increased risk of chronic diseases such as heart disease, type 2 diabetes, and colorectal cancer. It is recommended to consume red meat in moderation and choose lean cuts.

Poultry and Health

Poultry is a lean source of protein that is lower in saturated fat compared to red meat. It is also a good source of essential nutrients such as niacin, vitamin B6, and phosphorus. Skinless poultry is a healthier option as it reduces the intake of saturated fat.

Fish and Seafood and Health

Fish and seafood are excellent sources of high-quality protein and omega-3 fatty acids, which have been shown to support heart health, brain function, and reduce inflammation. Fatty fish such as salmon, mackerel, and sardines are particularly high in omega-3 fatty acids.

Dairy Products and Health

Dairy products provide high-quality protein along with calcium, vitamin D, and other essential nutrients. They support bone health, muscle function, and overall growth and development.

Low-fat and fat-free dairy options are recommended to reduce the intake of saturated fat.

Chapter 8: Plant Proteins

Nutritional Benefits

Plant proteins are lower in fat and calories compared to animal proteins and provide additional nutrients such as fiber, vitamins, and minerals. They are also more environmentally sustainable.

Common Plant Protein Sources

- Legumes: Beans, lentils, and peas are excellent sources of protein and fiber.

- Nuts and Seeds: These provide healthy fats along with protein.

- Whole Grains: Quinoa, brown rice, and oats contribute to protein intake and offer complex carbohydrates.

- Soy Products: Tofu, tempeh, and edamame are versatile sources of protein for vegetarians and vegans.

- Vegetables: Certain vegetables like broccoli and spinach also contribute to protein intake.

Health Considerations

Plant proteins are beneficial for overall health and can be part of a balanced diet. Combining different plant proteins ensures adequate intake of all essential amino acids.

Environmental Sustainability

Plant proteins have a lower environmental impact compared to animal proteins. They require less land, water, and energy to produce, making them a more sustainable choice.

Nutritional Advantages of Plant Proteins

1. Fiber: Plant proteins are rich in dietary fiber, which supports digestive health and reduces the risk of chronic diseases.

2. Phytochemicals: Plant proteins contain phytochemicals such as antioxidants that protect against cellular damage.

3. Low Saturated Fat: Plant proteins are typically low in saturated fat, reducing the risk of heart disease.

Complete Plant Protein Sources

Some plant foods are considered complete proteins because they contain all essential amino acids. These include:

- Quinoa: A gluten-free grain that provides complete protein and is rich in fiber and minerals.

- Soy Products: Tofu, tempeh, and edamame are complete protein sources and versatile ingredients in vegetarian and vegan diets.

- Buckwheat: A grain-like seed that offers complete protein and is high in antioxidants.

Combining Plant Proteins

Combining different plant proteins can provide a complete amino acid profile. Examples include:

- Rice and Beans: A classic combination that provides all essential amino acids.

- Hummus and Whole Wheat Bread: Chickpeas and whole wheat provide complementary amino acids.

- Peanut Butter and Oats: A combination of legumes and grains that delivers complete protein.

Plant Protein Supplements

Plant-based protein supplements such as pea protein, hemp protein, and brown rice protein are popular alternatives to animal-based supplements. They are suitable for individuals with dietary restrictions or allergies.

Cooking with Plant Proteins

Incorporating plant proteins into meals can be easy and delicious. Examples include:

- Bean and Lentil Stews: Hearty and protein-rich.

- Tofu Stir-Fries: Versatile and customizable with various vegetables and sauces.

- Nut and Seed Butters: Spread on whole grain bread or added to smoothies for a protein boost.

Chapter 9: Protein Needs and Recommendations

Daily Protein Requirements

Protein needs vary based on age, gender,

weight, and activity level. The Recommended Dietary Allowance (RDA) for protein is 0.8 grams per kilogram of body weight for adults. For children, the needs are higher relative to their body weight to support growth and development.

Protein Needs for Different Age Groups

- Infants (0-6 months): 1.52g/kg

- Infants (7-12 months): 1.2g/kg

- Children (1-3 years): 1.05g/kg

- Children (4-8 years): 0.95g/kg

- Children (9-13 years): 0.95g/kg

- Teens (14-18 years): Boys need about 52 grams, and girls need about 46 grams of protein per day.

- Adults (19 years and older): 0.8g/kg

- Older Adults (65 years and older): 1.0-1.2g/kg

Calculating Protein Needs

To calculate your protein needs, multiply your weight in kilograms by the recommended grams of protein per kilogram. For example, a 10-year-old child weighing 30 kilograms needs 0.95 grams of protein per kilogram:

- 30 kg x 0.95 g/kg = 28.5 grams of protein per day.

Protein Needs for Special Populations

Certain populations may have higher protein needs, including:

- Athletes: Increased protein intake is needed to support muscle repair and growth.

- Pregnant and Lactating Women: Additional protein is required to support fetal development and milk production.

- Older Adults: Higher protein intake helps prevent muscle loss and maintain functional independence.

- Individuals with Chronic Illness: Increased protein may be necessary for tissue repair and immune function.

Protein Timing

Distributing protein intake evenly throughout the day can optimize muscle protein synthesis. Consuming 20-30 grams of protein per meal is recommended for most adults. Including a source of protein in each meal and snack helps meet daily protein needs.

Protein Quality and Digestibility

High-quality proteins that are easily digestible and contain all essential amino acids should be prioritized. Animal proteins and certain plant proteins like soy and quinoa are considered high-quality proteins.

Protein in Different Dietary Patterns

- Omnivorous Diets: Include both animal and plant protein sources.

- Vegetarian Diets: Rely on plant proteins, dairy, and eggs.

- Vegan Diets: Exclusively plant-based protein sources.

Chapter 10: Protein in Daily Life

Incorporating Protein into Meals

Ensuring adequate protein intake throughout the day is essential for growth and development. Here are some tips for including protein in your daily meals:

Breakfast

- Eggs or Egg Whites: Scrambled, boiled, or in an omelet.

- Greek Yogurt with Fruit: High in protein and probiotics.

- Whole-Grain Toast with Peanut Butter: A quick and nutritious option.

- Smoothies with Protein Powder: Convenient and customizable.

Lunch

- Grilled Chicken or Turkey Sandwich: Lean protein on whole-grain bread.

- Salad with Beans or Tofu: Fresh vegetables with plant-based protein.

- Quinoa Bowl with Vegetables: Nutritious and satisfying.

- Lentil Soup: Rich in protein and fiber.

Dinner

- Baked Salmon or Chicken Breast: High-quality protein with healthy fats.

- Stir-Fry with Tofu and Vegetables: Versatile and nutritious.

- Black Bean Tacos: Plant-based protein in a flavorful dish.

- Pasta with Meat Sauce: Balanced with protein and carbohydrates.

Snacks

- Nuts and Seeds: Portable and protein-packed.

- String Cheese: Convenient and satisfying.

- Protein Bars: Ideal for on-the-go.

- Hummus with Vegetables: Nutritious and delicious.

Balancing Protein Intake

It's important to balance protein intake with other nutrients like carbohydrates and fats. A balanced diet ensures that you get all the vitamins and minerals needed for overall health.

Meal Planning and Preparation

Planning meals and snacks in advance can help ensure consistent protein intake. Batch cooking and preparing protein-rich foods in bulk can save time and provide convenient options throughout the week.

Hydration and Protein

Adequate hydration is essential when consuming a high-protein diet. Water helps with digestion, nutrient absorption, and the elimination of waste products from protein metabolism.

Protein and Physical Activity

Including protein in meals and snacks before and after exercise can support energy levels, muscle recovery, and overall performance. Combining protein with carbohydrates post-exercise can enhance glycogen replenishment and muscle repair.

Chapter 11: Protein in Different Life Stages

Protein Needs for Infants and Toddlers

Infants and toddlers require more protein relative to their body weight to support rapid growth and development. Breast milk and formula provide adequate protein for infants, while toddlers benefit from a variety of protein-rich foods.

Protein Needs for Children

Children need sufficient protein to support growth, muscle development, and immune function. Including a variety of protein sources in their diet ensures they receive all essential amino acids.

Protein Needs for Adolescents

During adolescence, protein needs increase to support the growth spurts and increased muscle mass associated with puberty. Active teens, especially athletes, may require additional protein.

Protein Needs for Adults

Adults need protein to maintain muscle mass, repair tissues, and support overall health. The RDA of 0.8 grams per kilogram of body weight is sufficient for most adults, but those who are physically active or have higher muscle mass may need more.

Protein Needs for Older Adults

Older adults may require more protein to prevent muscle loss and support overall health. The recommended intake is around 1.0-1.2 grams per kilogram of body weight to help maintain muscle mass and strength.

Protein Needs During Pregnancy and Lactation

Pregnant and lactating women require additional protein to support fetal development and milk production. The RDA for pregnant women is 1.1 grams per kilogram of body weight, and for lactating women, it is 1.3 grams per kilogram.

Protein Needs for Athletes

Athletes have higher protein needs to support muscle repair, recovery, and growth. The recommended intake varies based on the type and intensity of exercise, typically ranging from 1.2 to 2.0 grams per kilogram of body weight.

Protein Needs for Individuals with Chronic Illness

Individuals with chronic illnesses or injuries may require increased protein intake to support tissue repair, immune function, and overall recovery. A healthcare professional can provide personalized recommendations based on specific needs.

Chapter 12: Protein for Athletes

Importance of Protein for Athletes

Athletes have higher protein needs to support muscle repair, recovery, and growth. Protein helps in repairing damaged muscle fibers and promotes muscle protein synthesis after intense physical activity.

Protein Timing

Consuming protein after exercise is crucial for recovery. The anabolic window, or the period shortly after exercise, is when the body is most efficient at using protein to repair and build muscles. A protein-rich meal or snack within 30 minutes to two hours post-workout is beneficial.

Recommended Protein Intake for Athletes

- Endurance Athletes: 1.2-1.4 grams of protein per kilogram of body weight.

- Strength Athletes: 1.6-1.7 grams of protein per kilogram of body weight.

Protein Sources for Athletes

Athletes should focus on high-quality protein sources that provide all essential amino acids. Both animal and plant-based proteins can be effective when combined appropriately.

Pre-Workout Protein

Consuming a small amount of protein before exercise can help provide amino acids for muscle protein synthesis and reduce muscle breakdown during exercise. Examples include a protein shake, Greek yogurt, or a small serving of chicken or tofu.

Post-Workout Protein

Consuming protein after exercise is essential for muscle recovery and growth. Combining protein with carbohydrates can enhance glycogen replenishment and promote muscle repair. Examples include a protein shake with fruit, a chicken and vegetable stir-fry, or a smoothie with protein powder and banana.

Protein and Hydration

Staying hydrated is crucial for athletes, especially when consuming higher amounts of protein. Adequate water intake supports digestion, nutrient absorption, and the elimination of waste products from protein metabolism.

Protein Supplements for Athletes

Protein supplements such as whey protein, casein protein, and plant-based protein powders can be convenient options for athletes to meet their protein needs. It's important to choose high-quality supplements and use them as part of a balanced diet.

Protein and Injury Recovery

Increased protein intake is often recommended for athletes recovering from injuries to support tissue repair and healing. Including a variety of protein sources and distributing protein intake evenly throughout the day can optimize recovery.

Protein and Performance

Adequate protein intake supports athletic performance by promoting muscle strength, endurance, and recovery. Balancing protein with other nutrients such as carbohydrates and fats is essential for overall energy and performance.

Chapter 13: Cooking and Preparing Protein-Rich Foods

Cooking Techniques for Protein Foods

- Grilling: Ideal for meats and vegetables.

- Baking: Great for fish, poultry, and legumes.

- Stir-frying: Perfect for quick-cooking proteins like tofu and shrimp.

- Boiling: Suitable for eggs, beans, and grains.

- Steaming: Retains nutrients and flavor in vegetables and fish.

Healthy Protein Recipes

Recipe 1: Baked Salmon with Quinoa

- Ingredients: 2 salmon fillets, 1 cup quinoa, 2 cups water, 1 tablespoon olive oil, salt, pepper, lemon slices.

- Instructions:

1. Preheat oven to 375°F (190°C).

2. Season salmon fillets with olive oil, salt,and pepper.

3. Place salmon on a baking sheet and bake for 20-25 minutes.

4. In a saucepan, bring water to a boil. Add quinoa, reduce heat, and simmer for 15 minutes.

5. Serve baked salmon over quinoa with a squeeze of lemon.

Recipe 2: Lentil and Vegetable Stir-Fry

- Ingredients: 1 cup lentils, 2 cups water, 1 bell pepper, 1 zucchini, 1 cup broccoli, 2 tablespoons soy sauce, 1 tablespoon olive oil, garlic.

- Instructions:

1. Cook lentils in water until tender, about 20 minutes.

2. Heat olive oil in a pan, add garlic, and stir-fry vegetables until tender.

3. Add cooked lentils and soy sauce, stir well.

4. Serve hot.

Recipe 3: Greek Yogurt Parfait

- Ingredients: 1 cup Greek yogurt, 1/2 cup mixed berries, 1/4 cup granola, honey.

- Instructions:

1. Layer Greek yogurt, mixed berries, and granola in a glass.

2. Drizzle with honey.

3. Enjoy as a healthy breakfast or snack.

Recipe 4: Chicken and Vegetable Skewers

- Ingredients: 2 chicken breasts, 1 bell pepper, 1 zucchini, 1 red onion, 2 tablespoons olive oil, salt, pepper, paprika.

- Instructions:

1. Cut chicken and vegetables into bite-sized pieces.

2. Thread chicken and vegetables onto skewers.

3. Brush with olive oil and season with salt, pepper, and paprika.

4. Grill skewers over medium heat until chicken is cooked through and vegetables are tender.

Recipe 5: Black Bean and Quinoa Salad

- Ingredients: 1 cup cooked quinoa, 1 can black beans (drained and rinsed), 1 cup corn, 1 bell pepper (diced), 1 avocado (diced), 1/4 cup chopped cilantro, juice of 1 lime, 2 tablespoons olive oil, salt, pepper.

- Instructions:

1. In a large bowl, combine quinoa, black beans, corn, bell pepper, avocado, and cilantro.

2. In a small bowl, whisk together lime juice, olive oil, salt, and pepper.

3. Pour dressing over salad and toss to combine.

Healthy Cooking Tips

- Use healthy cooking methods like grilling, baking, and steaming.

- Avoid deep frying and excessive use of oils and fats.

- Season with herbs and spices instead of salt to enhance flavor without adding sodium.

- Include a variety of colorful vegetables in meals to boost nutrient intake.

- Prepare meals in advance to ensure healthy options are readily available.

Meal Planning and Preparation

Planning and preparing protein-rich meals in advance can help ensure consistent protein intake and support overall health. Batch cooking, meal prepping, and using leftovers creatively can save time and provide nutritious meals throughout the week.

Enhancing Flavor and Nutrition

- Marinating: Marinating meats and vegetables can enhance flavor and tenderize proteins.

- Herbs and Spices: Using herbs and spices can add flavor without extra calories or sodium.

- Healthy Fats: Incorporating healthy fats like olive oil, avocado, and nuts can improve the taste and nutritional value of meals.

Chapter 14: Protein Supplements

Types of Protein Supplements

- Whey Protein: A fast-digesting protein derived from milk, ideal for post-workout recovery.

- Casein Protein: A slow-digesting protein from milk, suitable for nighttime use.

- Soy Protein: A plant-based protein rich in essential amino acids.

- Pea Protein: A plant-based protein that's easy to digest and hypoallergenic.

- Hemp Protein: A plant-based protein with additional omega-3 fatty acids.

- Rice Protein: A plant-based protein that is hypoallergenic and easily digestible.

- Egg Protein: A high-quality protein derived from egg whites.

Benefits of Protein Supplements

Protein supplements can help meet daily protein requirements, support muscle recovery, and provide a convenient source of protein for busy individuals. They can be particularly beneficial for athletes, vegetarians, vegans, and those with increased protein needs.

How to Use Protein Supplements

Protein supplements can be mixed with water, milk, or blended into smoothies. They can also be added to recipes like oatmeal, pancakes, and baked goods for an extra protein boost.

Choosing the Right Protein Supplement

When selecting a protein supplement, consider factors like

protein content, ingredient quality, and dietary restrictions. It's also important to choose a supplement that fits your taste preferences and lifestyle.

Potential Side Effects and Considerations

While protein supplements are generally safe, excessive protein intake can strain the kidneys and liver. It's important to follow recommended dosages and consult with a healthcare professional if you have any underlying health conditions.

Comparing Protein Supplements

- Whey Protein: High in branched-chain amino acids (BCAAs), quickly absorbed, supports muscle recovery.

- Casein Protein: Slow-digesting, provides a sustained release of amino acids, ideal for nighttime use.

- Soy Protein: Plant-based, rich in essential amino acids, supports heart health.

- Pea Protein: Hypoallergenic, easy to digest, suitable for vegans and those with food allergies.

- Hemp Protein: Contains omega-3 fatty acids, fiber, and essential amino acids, supports overall health.

- Rice Protein: Hypoallergenic, easily digestible, suitable for those with food sensitivities.

- Egg Protein: Complete protein, high biological value, supports muscle growth and repair.

Protein Supplement Brands

- Optimum Nutrition: Known for high-quality whey protein supplements.

- Garden of Life: Offers organic plant-based protein powders.

- Vega: Provides a range of vegan protein supplements.

- Dymatize: Known for hydrolyzed whey protein and isolate supplements.

- Orgain: Offers organic protein powders suitable for vegetarians and vegans.

Incorporating Protein Supplements into Meals

- Smoothies: Blend protein powder with fruits, vegetables, and liquids for a nutritious meal.

- Baked Goods: Add protein powder to pancakes, muffins, and cookies for an extra protein boost.

- Oatmeal: Stir protein powder into oatmeal or overnight oats for a protein-rich breakfast.

- Yogurt: Mix protein powder into Greek yogurt for a high-protein snack.

Chapter 15: Protein and Weight Management

Protein and Satiety

Protein promotes satiety, which helps control appetite and reduce overall calorie intake. Including protein in meals and snacks can help prevent overeating and support weight management.

Thermic Effect of Protein

Protein has a higher thermic effect compared to carbohydrates and fats, meaning the body uses more energy to digest and metabolize protein. This increased energy expenditure can support weight loss and weight management.

Protein and Muscle Mass

Maintaining or increasing muscle mass through adequate protein intake can boost metabolism and support weight management. Muscle tissue burns more calories at rest compared to fat tissue, contributing to a higher metabolic rate.

High-Protein Diets for Weight Loss

High-protein diets can be effective for weight loss by promoting satiety, preserving muscle mass, and increasing energy expenditure. Examples of high-protein diets include the Atkins diet, the Dukan diet, and the ketogenic diet.

Balanced Approach to Weight Management

While high-protein diets can be beneficial, it's important to balance protein intake with other nutrients such as carbohydrates and fats. A balanced diet that includes a variety of foods can support overall health and sustainable weight management.

Meal Planning for Weight Management

Planning and preparing balanced meals that include protein, carbohydrates, and healthy fats can help support weight management goals. Portion control and mindful eating are also important strategies.

Protein-Rich Foods for Weight Management

- Lean Meats: Chicken breast, turkey, lean beef.

- Fish and Seafood: Salmon, tuna, shrimp.

- Eggs: Whole eggs and egg whites.

- Dairy: Greek yogurt, cottage cheese, low-fat milk.

- Legumes: Lentils, black beans, chickpeas.

- Nuts and Seeds: Almonds, peanuts, chia seeds.

- Soy Products: Tofu, tempeh, edamame.

- Whole Grains: Quinoa, brown rice, oats.

Combining Protein with Fiber

Combining protein with fiber-rich foods can enhance satiety and support weight management. Examples include:

- Salads with Beans and Vegetables: High in fiber and protein.

- Greek Yogurt with Berries: Combines protein and fiber.

- Lentil Soup with Vegetables: Nutrient-dense and filling.

Protein Snacks for Weight Management

- Hard-Boiled Eggs: Portable and protein-rich.

- String Cheese: Convenient and satisfying.

- Protein Bars: Ideal for on-the-go.

- Hummus with Carrot Sticks: Nutritious and delicious.

- Almonds: High in protein and healthy fats.

Chapter 16: Protein and Chronic Diseases

Protein and Heart Health

Consuming high-quality protein sources, such as fish, lean meats, and plant-based proteins, can support heart health. Omega-3 fatty acids found in fatty fish have been shown to reduce the risk of heart disease. Plant-based proteins can also lower cholesterol levels and improve cardiovascular health.

Protein and Diabetes Management

Protein can help regulate blood sugar levels and support diabetes management. Including protein in meals and snacks can slow the absorption of carbohydrates and prevent blood sugar spikes. Lean meats, fish, eggs, and plant-based proteins are good choices for individuals with diabetes.

Protein and Kidney Health

While high-protein diets are generally safe for healthy individuals, those with kidney disease may need to limit their protein intake to prevent further kidney damage. It's important for individuals with kidney conditions to work with a healthcare professional to determine appropriate protein intake.

Protein and Bone Health

Protein plays a crucial role in maintaining bone health by supporting bone density and strength. Adequate protein intake, along with calcium and vitamin D, is essential for preventing osteoporosis and fractures, especially in older adults.

Protein and Cancer

Research on the relationship between protein intake and cancer risk is ongoing. Some studies suggest that high intake of red and processed meats may increase the risk of certain cancers, while plant-based proteins may have a protective effect. A balanced diet that includes a variety of protein sources is recommended.

Protein and Weight Management

As discussed in Chapter 15, protein supports weight management by promoting satiety, preserving muscle mass, and increasing energy expenditure. Maintaining a healthy weight is crucial for reducing the risk of chronic diseases such as heart disease, diabetes, and certain cancers.

Protein and Immune Function

Protein is essential for a healthy immune system. It supports the production of antibodies and immune cells that protect the body from infections. Adequate protein intake is important for overall immune function and resilience against illnesses.

Protein and Digestive Health

Protein supports digestive health by providing the building blocks for enzymes involved in digestion. Additionally, certain protein-rich foods, such as yogurt and kefir, contain probiotics that promote gut health.

Balancing Protein Intake with Chronic Disease Management

Balancing protein intake with other nutrients and considering individual health conditions is essential for managing chronic diseases. Working with a healthcare professional or registered dietitian can help develop a personalized nutrition plan.

Chapter 17: Common Myths About Protein

Myth 1: High-Protein Diets Are Bad for Your Kidneys

Fact: For healthy individuals, high-protein diets do not harm kidney function. However, those with pre-existing kidney conditions should consult a healthcare professional.

Myth 2: More Protein Means More Muscle

Fact: While protein is essential for muscle growth, simply eating more protein will not result in increased muscle mass without proper exercise and training.

Myth 3: Plant Proteins Are Inferior to Animal Proteins

Fact: Plant proteins can provide all essential amino acids when consumed in a varied and balanced diet. They also offer additional health benefits like fiber and antioxidants.

Myth 4: You Can Only Absorb a Certain Amount of Protein at Once

Fact: The body can utilize protein efficiently throughout the day, and there is no fixed limit on how much protein can be absorbed in one meal. However, spreading protein intake across meals may optimize muscle protein synthesis.

Myth 5: Protein Causes Weight Gain

Fact: Protein itself does not cause weight gain. Weight gain occurs when there is a caloric surplus. Protein can aid in weight management by promoting satiety and supporting muscle mass.

Myth 6: All Protein Supplements Are the Same

Fact: Protein supplements vary in terms of protein content, amino acid profile, digestibility, and ingredient quality. It's important to choose a high-quality supplement that fits individual needs and preferences.

Myth 7: You Need Protein Immediately After a Workout

Fact: While consuming protein after a workout is beneficial for muscle recovery, the anabolic window is not as short as previously thought. Consuming protein within a few hours post-workout is generally sufficient.

Myth 8: High-Protein Diets Are Only for Bodybuilders

Fact: High-protein diets can benefit a wide range of individuals, including athletes, older adults, and those looking to manage their weight or support overall health.

Myth 9: Protein-Rich Diets Are Difficult to Follow

Fact: Incorporating protein-rich foods into meals and snacks can be simple and convenient. There are many delicious and nutritious protein sources available to suit different dietary preferences.

Myth 10: Protein Shakes Are Necessary for Muscle Gain

Fact: While protein shakes can be a convenient way to meet protein needs, they are not necessary for muscle gain. Whole food sources of protein can also effectively support muscle growth and recovery.

Chapter 18: The Future of Protein

Innovations in Protein Sources

- Lab-Grown Meat: Cultured meat produced from animal cells offers a sustainable alternative to traditional meat.

- Insect Protein: Insects like crickets and mealworms are high in protein and environmentally friendly.

- Algae Protein: Algae and seaweed are being explored as new sources of protein with potential health benefits.

- Fungal Protein: Mycoprotein, derived from fungi, is a sustainable and nutritious protein source.

Sustainability and Protein Production

With growing concerns about environmental impact, sustainable protein sources are becoming increasingly important. Reducing meat consumption and incorporating plant-based proteins can help lower the carbon footprint.

Technological Advancements

Advancements in biotechnology and food science are paving the way for innovative protein sources. These technologies aim to create sustainable, nutritious, and affordable protein options for the global population.

Personalized Nutrition and Protein

Personalized nutrition, guided by genetic testing and biomarkers, can help individuals optimize their protein intake based on their unique needs and health goals. This approach can enhance health outcomes and prevent chronic diseases.

Protein Fortification

Fortifying staple foods with protein can help address protein deficiency in populations with limited access to diverse protein sources. Protein fortification can improve nutritional status and support overall health.

Global Protein Trends

The demand for protein is increasing worldwide, driven by population growth and rising incomes. Meeting this demand sustainably requires innovative solutions and a shift towards more plant-based and alternative protein sources.

Ethical Considerations

The ethical implications of protein production, including animal welfare and environmental sustainability, are important factors shaping the future of protein. Ethical consumerism is driving demand for humane and sustainable protein options.

Protein and Public Health

Public health initiatives aimed at improving protein intake and promoting balanced diets can help address malnutrition and prevent diet-related chronic diseases. Education and awareness campaigns are essential for promoting healthy protein choices.

Chapter 19: Conclusion

The Importance of Protein

Protein is a crucial nutrient that supports growth, repair, and overall health. Understanding its sources, benefits, and requirements can help ensure you maintain a balanced and nutritious diet.

Encouragement to Explore

Explore different protein sources and find what works best for you. Balance your diet with a variety of foods to meet your nutritional needs and support a healthy lifestyle.

Final Thoughts

By incorporating a variety of protein-rich foods into your diet, you can ensure that your body gets the essential nutrients it needs to function optimally. Remember to consider both animal and plant-based protein sources and choose options that align with your health goals and environmental values.

Chapter 20: Glossary

Amino Acids

The building blocks of proteins.

Complete Proteins

Proteins that contain all essential amino acids.

Incomplete Proteins

Proteins that lack one or more essential amino acids.

Essential Amino Acids

Amino acids that must be obtained from the diet.

Non-Essential Amino Acids

Amino acids that can be synthesized by the body.

Conditional Amino Acids

Amino acids that are usually not essential except in times of illness and stress.

Bioavailability

The extent to which nutrients can be absorbed and utilized by the body.

Complementary Proteins

Combining two or more incomplete protein sources to provide all essential amino acids.

Biological Value (BV)

A measure of the proportion of absorbed protein that becomes incorporated into the proteins of the organism's body.

Net Protein Utilization (NPU)

A measure of the percentage of dietary protein that is retained in the body for growth and maintenance.

Protein Digestibility-Corrected Amino Acid Score (PDCAAS)

A method used to evaluate the protein quality of food based on its amino acid composition and digestibility.

Enzymes

Proteins that catalyze biochemical reactions.

Hormones

Regulatory proteins that control physiological processes.

Antibodies

Proteins that protect the body from pathogens.

Proteomics

The large-scale study of proteins.

Lab-Grown Meat

Cultured meat produced from animal cells.

Insect Protein

Protein derived from insects.

Algae Protein

Protein derived from algae and seaweed.

Fungal Protein

Protein derived from fungi, such as mycoprotein.

Chapter 21: Recommended Reading and Resources

Books

- "Good Enough to Eat: A Kid's Guide to Food and Nutrition" by Lizzy Rockwell

- "The Omnivore's Dilemma: Young Readers Edition" by Michael Pollan

- "Super Foods for Super Kids Cookbook" by Noelle Martin, Julie Stephenson, and Nicole Berring

- "Protein Power: The High-Protein/Low-Carbohydrate Way to Lose Weight, Feel Fit, and Boost Your Health—in Just Weeks!" by Michael R. Eades and Mary Dan Eades

- "The Plant-Based Athlete: A Game-Changing Approach to Peak Performance" by Matt Frazier and Robert Cheeke

Websites

- [ChooseMyPlate.gov](https://www.choosemyplate.gov/)

- [Nutrition.gov](https://www.nutrition.gov/)

- [EatRight.org](https://www.eatright.org/)

- [American Society for Nutrition](https://nutrition.org/)

- [Protein Research Foundation](https://www.proteinresearchfoundation.org/)

Journals and Articles

- "Journal of Nutrition"

- "American Journal of Clinical Nutrition"

- "Nutrition Reviews"

- "Annual Review of Nutrition"

Research Databases

- PubMed

- Google Scholar

- ScienceDirect

Online Courses

- "Nutrition and Health: Macronutrients and Overnutrition" by Wageningen University on edX

- "Introduction to Human Nutrition" by Stanford University on Coursera

- "Sports and Exercise Nutrition" by The Open University on FutureLearn